THRIVE & SHINE, YOUR DAILY WELLNESS JOURNAL

Transforming Stress into Strength,
One Day at a Time

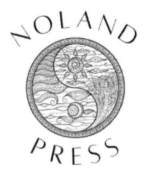

Joshua D. Noland

JoshNoland.com

THRIVE & SHINE, YOUR DAILY WELLNESS JOURNAL

Transforming Stress into Strength, One Day at a Time

Joshua D. Noland

Copyright © 2025 Joshua D. Noland

ISBN: 978-1-965040-06-5

All Rights Reserved. No part of this publication may be reproduced, distributed, or transmitted in any form or by any means, including photocopying, recording, or other electronic or mechanical methods, without the prior written permission from the author, except in the case of brief quotations embodied in critical reviews and certain other non-commercial uses permitted by copyright law.

The information given in this book should not be treated as a substitute for professional medical or clinical advice; always consult a medical or clinical practitioner. Any use of information in this book is at the reader's discretion and risk. Neither the author nor the publisher can be held responsible for any loss, claim, or damage arising from the use or misuse of the suggestions made.

Why You Need This Journal

This journal provides a structured approach to committing to your well-being, which is essential for leading a long, fulfilling life. By journaling daily, you'll create an optimistic outlook on life that goes a long way toward creating a positive mindset. Whether you want to lose weight, overcome common lifestyle diseases, or feel more energized, this journal will help you reflect on your choices, assess what's working, and recalibrate as needed, ensuring you're always moving forward, one step at a time.

This journal addresses the mental and emotional aspects of wellness. Daily gratitude practice, positive affirmations, and reflecting on your progress will help you develop a positive mindset, reduce stress, and recognize the progress you're making. Over time, these tiny changes accumulate to produce powerful results: an improved mood, better relationships with yourself and others, and a stronger sense of purpose. In other words, by using this journal regularly, you'll build a healthier lifestyle from the inside out, safeguarding both your short-term vitality and long-term well-being.

Created by Someone Who Transformed Their Health Using These Modalities

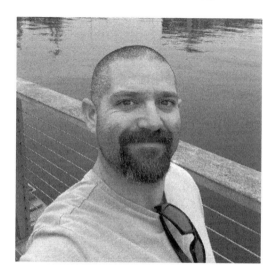

Joshua D. Noland is a Holistic Lifestyle Strategist, author, and host of the Health Unfiltered podcast. His passion is helping people overcome their health struggles by teaching them how to develop mental wellness, enabling them to live their lives to the fullest. He was able to lose over eighty pounds and keep it off, in addition to overcoming IBS, food addiction, and depression. Joshua is also an avid outdoorsman and a devoted dog father, continually inspired by nature and his loyal canine companions. Visit **JoshNoland.com** to learn more about him and explore his extensive collection of works.

Your Wellness Intentions

Use this page to set your intentions for this journal and add your contact information in case you lose it.

Name: _____

Phone Number: _____

What do you hope to achieve by keeping a daily journal?

_____
_____
_____
_____
_____
_____
_____

The reasons you decide to improve your health will be crucial when you become discouraged or unmotivated to continue working on yourself. Whenever this happens, come back to this page and reflect on the answer you provided.

Put yourself back in the headspace you were in when you first started and reflect on these feelings. This will help you carry on and stay consistent with your journaling journey.

Within this journal, you'll find concise summaries of the modalities utilized to transform stress into strengths.

Want to dive deeper and explore the full benefits?

Visit <u>LaunchYourEvolution.com</u> for informative articles, recipes, and much more!

INTRODUCTION

Your mental wellness is arguably the most critical part of your overall health. After all, if you're stressed, depressed, or anxious, you'll be less likely to get enough quality sleep, exercise, or eat the foods that will make you feel and look your best. These concepts of wellness are interconnected, and they begin with cultivating a positive mindset.

When you are motivated to eat to fuel your body rather than for emotional support, you are in the right mindset.

Exercise can take on a very different form for different individuals. For some, simply going for walks is enough at first; then, you can gradually incorporate strength training, which is essential for maintaining bone health, performing everyday tasks with strength, and more. No matter what's right for you, the most important thing is to find something you don't mind doing and stick with it long enough to see results.

Cultivating a positive mindset involves more than exercise and a balanced diet. Getting quality sleep and staying hydrated are also vital pieces of the puzzle. That's why these key areas have also been included in this journal. By taking small steps each day, you'll start to see significant changes over time.

Remember, a holistic approach to health involves caring for both your body and your mind. This journal will guide you in setting intentions, practicing gratitude, and reflecting on your progress so you can begin to feel better, inside and out.

THE FIVE PILLARS OF OPTIMAL HEALTH

Focusing on mental wellness, sleep, fitness, hydration, and proper nutrition are key factors that will have the most significant impact on your health. That is why they are featured in this journal. If you can incorporate filling out this journal into your daily routine, your mental health will improve, and subsequently, all the other aspects will improve as a result.

Mental Wellness

A balanced mind is crucial for managing stress, maintaining motivation, regulating emotions, and developing resilience. Prioritizing mental health can enhance self-esteem, foster stronger relationships, and lead to greater overall life satisfaction.

Today I feel

Tracking your mood can help you dial in what is making the biggest impact on your feelings. This can significantly impact your motivation to focus on your fitness and diet. Your thought patterns and activity level can impact your mood. Track it so you can go back and determine what made you feel that way on a particular day.

I am grateful for

Gratitude is the recognition and appreciation of the positive aspects of your life, both big and small. It's important because it shifts your focus from what you lack to what you already have, fostering a more optimistic mindset and reducing stress. A consistent gratitude practice can deepen relationships, boost emotional resilience, and help you navigate challenges with a more positive outlook.

Affirmations

Positive affirmations are short, uplifting statements that you repeat to yourself daily to cultivate self-belief and a more optimistic mindset. This is important because reciting positive affirmations aloud can help to counteract negative self-talk, boost self-esteem, and reinforce a sense of confidence and resilience. By consistently reminding yourself of your worth, capabilities, and potential, you can shift your inner dialogue and shape how you view challenges and setbacks.

Thoughts & Reflections

Writing down your thoughts and reflections daily helps you process emotions, appreciate your successes, identify patterns, and learn from experiences, thereby enhancing mental clarity and emotional resilience. This practice also reduces stress and anxiety, ultimately leading to improved physical health.

Sleep

Adequate rest is vital for physical repair, mental processing, and emotional regulation. Quality sleep improves cognitive function, mood, and overall well-being, making it a cornerstone of wellness. Most people require 7 to 9 hours of quality sleep each night.

Getting the right amount of quality sleep could easily be the most crucial aspect of overall health due to its impact on all the other pillars of optimal health.

Previous night's sleep quality

Keeping a log of how many hours and the quality of your sleep can help you recognize the connection between getting proper rest and how you feel.

Fitness

Being physically active supports optimal health by boosting cardiovascular function, strengthening muscles and bones, and maintaining a healthy weight. It also reduces stress, improves mood, and helps prevent chronic diseases, making regular movement a crucial part of any wellness routine.

Fitness log

Tracking your activity level can help you see if you are meeting your exercise goals or not. It's beneficial to know what you have done, as it will give you a sense of accomplishment.

Hydration

Hydration is essential for numerous bodily functions, including regulating body temperature, maintaining joint lubrication, and ensuring the proper functioning of organs. It also supports digestion, helps flush out toxins, and maintain energy levels, making it a simple yet powerful way to boost overall health and well-being. Electrolytes are also a crucial factor in maintaining proper hydration.

Water Tracker

It's commonly recommended to drink eight 8-ounce glasses (roughly 2 liters) of water a day. However, individual needs vary based on factors like activity level, climate, and overall health. Staying attuned to your thirst and aiming for clear or light-colored urine are good indicators that you're staying adequately hydrated. You may need to supplement your water with electrolytes if you are not getting enough from your diet.

Proper Nutrition

A nutrient-dense diet of whole foods provides the body with essential vitamins, minerals, and energy. It supports healthy bodily functions, helps manage weight, and reduces the risk of chronic diseases. I recommend focusing on eating whole foods, especially protein and fat from animal sources, and limiting carbs as much as possible.

Food Log

It's hard to remember what you ate yesterday, let alone what you ate at the beginning of the week. Make the process of tracking your nutrition bulletproof by writing down everything you eat and drink so you can discover what foods make you feel good and which ones make you feel shitty. Your diet can affect you physically and mentally.

Personalize your journal by using stickers, drawings, or different colored pens to make it truly yours and more enjoyable.

HOW TO ESTABLISH A CONSISTENT JOURNALING ROUTINE

1. Start Small (Seriously, Tiny)

Don't try to write an essay every day. Start with just one sentence. Something like

"Today I felt ___ because ___."

Once that feels easy, you'll naturally want to write more.

2. Pick a Time You Can Stick To

Consistency over perfection. Try attaching journaling to something you already do.

I find that setting intentions and writing/ reciting positive affirmations in the morning followed by writing down my thoughts and reflections in the evenings works best for me. However, it's essential to determine what works best for you and your schedule.

3. Keep It Private, Keep It Real

Don't censor yourself. This is for you, not Instagram. The more honest you are, the more therapeutic this process becomes.

4. Set a Reminder or Habit Stack

Use a calendar or phone reminder to prompt you to journal, or link journaling to another habit, such as: "After I pour my coffee, I write for 2 minutes."

5. Celebrate Wins

Each time you journal, give yourself a little dopamine boost. Say, "I did it." Check it off your to-do list and let yourself feel that little victory.

HOW TO USE THIS JOURNAL

This journal has been designed to be intuitive; however, if you would like to see examples or suggestions on how to utilize each section effectively, read on. If not, skip this section and start journaling now!

Today I feel

Circle the emotion that best identifies how you feel. This can be done first thing in the morning or later in the day to capture your overall mood for the day.

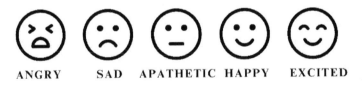

Use the section provided to the right of the visual representations to expand on how you are feeling and why you might be feeling this way.

Previous night's sleep quality

Consider the quality and amount of sleep you got the night before. Circle the smiley face if you got enough quality sleep or the sad face if you did not.

Fitness log

You have several options for utilizing this section.

1. Record the physical activities you participated in that day.
2. Log your physical activities as you do them.
3. Write down your fitness goals for the day and check them off as you accomplish them.

This can include your step count, strength training, cardiovascular exercise, stretching, mobility practices, or play. As long as you move your body, it counts.

Water Tracker

Cross off one water drop every time you drink eight ounces of water.

Suppose you use a larger water bottle, for example, a 32-ounce Hydroflask. You can check off four drops every time you finish it.

Food Log

Write down EVERYTHING you eat and drink before you consume it, or take a picture of it and log it later in the day. Try to estimate how much of each item you consumed for more accurate tracking.

I am grateful for

Write down three to five things you are grateful for. These could be things, people, situations, or anything else you are thankful to have in your life.

Affirmations

Write down three to five short, uplifting statements that you would like your subconscious to believe. Repeat each of these statements aloud three times.

Thoughts & Reflections

Write down anything you like in this section.

- What's on your mind at the moment?
- Something that stood out or felt meaningful today.
- A worry, doubt, or challenge you're facing.
- A random idea or insight that came to you.
- A decision you're trying to make.
- What went well today, and why?
- What didn't go as planned, and what did you learn from it?
- How did you respond to stress, and would you change anything?
- Did you notice any patterns in your behavior or emotions?
- Are you proud of something you did today?

Sample Pages

The following pages can help you get an idea of how you can use this journal. Just because this journal has been designed in a certain way doesn't mean you must follow it strictly. Feel free to mix it up and make it fit you and your style. Everyone thinks differently, and you must do what works best for you to maximize your progress.

DATE May, 18th 2025

TODAY I FEEL:

I woke up feeling lousy, so I meditated and had some coffee, which helped me feel better.

PREVIOUS NIGHT'S SLEEP QUALITY:

 8 HOURS

FITNESS LOG:

3min Cold Plunge, 5 min Warm Up
10 Squats, 10 Rows, 10 Chest flies, 10 Dead lifts,
10 Bicep curls, 10 Tricep straight arm pull downs, and
10 Lateral raises with bands.
10 leg raises, 2 min plank

WATER TRACKER:

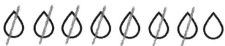

FOOD LOG:

BREAKFAST: 4 whole eggs and a 6 oz ribeye steak

LUNCH: Rotisserie chicken 1 leg 1 thigh and 1 wing

DINNER: 8 oz of pork belly, 1 oz queso fresco

SNACKS: 4 oz of beef jerky, 1 green apple, 1/2 of a papaya

DRINKS: 1 cup of coffee with 2 Tbls of heavy cream
12 oz can coke zero

I AM GRATEFUL FOR:

My health
New opportunities
My friends and family
Nature

AFFIRMATIONS:

I am going to have a great day!
I am worthy of love!
I am intelligent and kind!
Every day and in every way, I am better, better, and better!

THOUGHTS & REFLECTIONS:

I felt shitty when I first woke up, not sure why, but I meditated while my coffee was brewing and, after a few sips, I started feeling better.
I don't know what it is about this journal, but on the days I fill it out, I just feel good. I haven't been sticking with it every day, but I will make an additional effort this week to fill out my journal every day.
I did well on drinking water today and almost hit my goal.
Had a great workout. Damn, I hate getting into the cold plunge, but I feel so incredible when I get out.
I took my wife out on a dinner date this evening, and it was so nice to take a few hours just for us to catch up and not worry about anything.

"The past is history.
The future is a mystery.
Today is a gift.
That's why it's called the present."

Your Journey Awaits

Before you dive in, take a moment to acknowledge the commitment you're making to yourself by using this journal. You've already taken an important first step toward living a more balanced life. As you turn the pages ahead, remember that meaningful change doesn't happen overnight; it's built one day at a time. Be patient with yourself, celebrate every small victory, and keep your eyes on the bigger picture. You're not just filling out a journal; you're creating the foundation for a brighter, healthier future. Embrace this journey, trust the process, and know that each page you complete is a powerful step toward the life you deserve.

DATE _____

TODAY I FEEL:

😫 🙁 😐 🙂 😊 _____
                  _____
                  _____

PREVIOUS NIGHT'S SLEEP QUALITY:

🙁 🙂 _____ HOURS

FITNESS LOG:
_____
_____
_____
_____
_____

WATER TRACKER:

◯ ◯ ◯ ◯ ◯ ◯ ◯

FOOD LOG:

BREAKFAST: _____

LUNCH: _____

DINNER: _____

SNACKS: _____

DRINKS: _____

I AM GRATEFUL FOR:

_____
_____
_____
_____

AFFIRMATIONS:

_____
_____
_____
_____

THOUGHTS & REFLECTIONS:

_____
_____
_____
_____
_____
_____
_____
_____
_____
_____
_____

DATE _____

TODAY I FEEL:

😣 🙁 😐 🙂 😊   _____
_____
_____

PREVIOUS NIGHT'S SLEEP QUALITY:

🙁 🙂 _____ HOURS

FITNESS LOG:
_____
_____
_____
_____
_____

WATER TRACKER:

💧 💧 💧 💧 💧 💧 💧

FOOD LOG:

BREAKFAST:
_____

LUNCH:
_____

DINNER:
_____

SNACKS:
_____

DRINKS:
_____

I AM GRATEFUL FOR:

AFFIRMATIONS:

THOUGHTS & REFLECTIONS:

DATE_____

TODAY I FEEL:

😣 🙁 😐 🙂 😊 _____

PREVIOUS NIGHT'S SLEEP QUALITY:

🙁 🙂 _____ HOURS

FITNESS LOG:
_____
_____
_____
_____
_____

WATER TRACKER:

💧 💧 💧 💧 💧 💧 💧

FOOD LOG:

BREAKFAST:
_____

LUNCH:
_____

DINNER:
_____

SNACKS:
_____

DRINKS:
_____

I AM GRATEFUL FOR:

AFFIRMATIONS:

THOUGHTS & REFLECTIONS:

DATE_____

TODAY I FEEL:

😣 🙁 😐 🙂 😊 _____

PREVIOUS NIGHT'S SLEEP QUALITY:

🙁 🙂 _____ HOURS

FITNESS LOG:

_____
_____
_____
_____

WATER TRACKER:

💧💧💧💧💧💧💧

FOOD LOG:

BREAKFAST:
_____

LUNCH:
_____

DINNER:
_____

SNACKS:
_____

DRINKS:
_____

I AM GRATEFUL FOR:

_____
_____
_____
_____
_____

AFFIRMATIONS:

_____
_____
_____
_____

THOUGHTS & REFLECTIONS:

_____
_____
_____
_____
_____
_____
_____
_____
_____
_____
_____
_____
_____

DATE_____

TODAY I FEEL:

😣 🙁 😐 🙂 😊 _____

PREVIOUS NIGHT'S SLEEP QUALITY:

🙁 🙂 _____ HOURS

FITNESS LOG:

_____
_____
_____
_____

WATER TRACKER:

💧 💧 💧 💧 💧 💧 💧

FOOD LOG:

BREAKFAST:

LUNCH:

DINNER:

SNACKS:

DRINKS:

I AM GRATEFUL FOR:

AFFIRMATIONS:

THOUGHTS & REFLECTIONS:

DATE_____

TODAY I FEEL:

😣 🙁 😐 🙂 😊 _____
_____
_____
_____

PREVIOUS NIGHT'S SLEEP QUALITY:

🙁 🙂 _____ HOURS

FITNESS LOG:
_____
_____
_____
_____
_____

WATER TRACKER:

💧💧💧💧💧💧💧

FOOD LOG:

BREAKFAST:
_____

LUNCH:
_____

DINNER:
_____

SNACKS:
_____

DRINKS:
_____

I AM GRATEFUL FOR:

_____
_____
_____
_____

AFFIRMATIONS:

_____
_____
_____
_____

THOUGHTS & REFLECTIONS:

_____
_____
_____
_____
_____
_____
_____
_____
_____
_____
_____
_____

DATE_____

TODAY I FEEL:

😣 ☹️ 😐 🙂 😊 _____

PREVIOUS NIGHT'S SLEEP QUALITY:

☹️ 🙂 _____ HOURS

FITNESS LOG:

_____
_____
_____
_____

WATER TRACKER:

💧💧💧💧💧💧💧

FOOD LOG:

BREAKFAST:
_____

LUNCH:
_____

DINNER:
_____

SNACKS:
_____

DRINKS:
_____

I AM GRATEFUL FOR:

_____
_____
_____
_____

AFFIRMATIONS:

_____
_____
_____
_____

THOUGHTS & REFLECTIONS:

_____
_____
_____
_____
_____
_____
_____
_____
_____
_____
_____

DATE_____

TODAY I FEEL:

😖 ☹️ 😐 🙂 😊 _____
_____
_____

PREVIOUS NIGHT'S SLEEP QUALITY:

☹️ 🙂 _____ HOURS

FITNESS LOG:
_____
_____
_____
_____
_____

WATER TRACKER:
💧💧💧💧💧💧💧

FOOD LOG:

BREAKFAST:
_____

LUNCH:
_____

DINNER:
_____

SNACKS:
_____

DRINKS:
_____

I AM GRATEFUL FOR:

_____
_____
_____
_____
_____

AFFIRMATIONS:

_____
_____
_____
_____
_____

THOUGHTS & REFLECTIONS:

_____
_____
_____
_____
_____
_____
_____
_____
_____
_____
_____
_____
_____
_____

DATE_____

TODAY I FEEL:

😖 ☹️ 😐 🙂 😊 _____
_____
_____

PREVIOUS NIGHT'S SLEEP QUALITY:

☹️ 🙂 _____ HOURS

FITNESS LOG:

_____
_____
_____
_____
_____

WATER TRACKER:

💧💧💧💧💧💧💧

FOOD LOG:

BREAKFAST:
_____

LUNCH:
_____

DINNER:
_____

SNACKS:
_____

DRINKS:
_____

I AM GRATEFUL FOR:

AFFIRMATIONS:

THOUGHTS & REFLECTIONS:

DATE_____

TODAY I FEEL:

😣 ☹️ 😐 🙂 😊 _____
_____
_____

PREVIOUS NIGHT'S SLEEP QUALITY:

☹️ 🙂 _____ HOURS

FITNESS LOG:
_____
_____
_____
_____
_____

WATER TRACKER:

💧💧💧💧💧💧💧

FOOD LOG:

BREAKFAST:
_____

LUNCH:
_____

DINNER:
_____

SNACKS:
_____

DRINKS:
_____

I AM GRATEFUL FOR:

AFFIRMATIONS:

THOUGHTS & REFLECTIONS:

DATE_____

TODAY I FEEL:

😣 ☹️ 😐 🙂 😊

PREVIOUS NIGHT'S SLEEP QUALITY:

☹️ 🙂 _____ HOURS

FITNESS LOG:

WATER TRACKER:

💧💧💧💧💧💧💧

FOOD LOG:

BREAKFAST:

LUNCH:

DINNER:

SNACKS:

DRINKS:

I AM GRATEFUL FOR:

AFFIRMATIONS:

THOUGHTS & REFLECTIONS:

DATE _____

TODAY I FEEL:

😣 😕 😐 🙂 😊   _____
_____
_____

PREVIOUS NIGHT'S SLEEP QUALITY:

☹️ 🙂   _____ HOURS

FITNESS LOG:

_____
_____
_____
_____
_____

WATER TRACKER:

💧 💧 💧 💧 💧 💧 💧

FOOD LOG:

BREAKFAST: _____

LUNCH: _____

DINNER: _____

SNACKS: _____

DRINKS: _____

I AM GRATEFUL FOR:

AFFIRMATIONS:

THOUGHTS & REFLECTIONS:

DATE_____

TODAY I FEEL:

😣 ☹️ 😐 🙂 😊 _____

PREVIOUS NIGHT'S SLEEP QUALITY:

☹️ 🙂 _____ HOURS

FITNESS LOG:

_____
_____
_____
_____
_____

WATER TRACKER:

○ ○ ○ ○ ○ ○ ○

FOOD LOG:

BREAKFAST:
_____

LUNCH:
_____

DINNER:
_____

SNACKS:
_____

DRINKS:
_____

I AM GRATEFUL FOR:

_____
_____
_____
_____
_____

AFFIRMATIONS:

_____
_____
_____
_____

THOUGHTS & REFLECTIONS:

_____
_____
_____
_____
_____
_____
_____
_____
_____
_____
_____
_____
_____

DATE_____

TODAY I FEEL:

😫 ☹️ 😐 🙂 😊 _____

PREVIOUS NIGHT'S SLEEP QUALITY:

☹️ 🙂 _____ HOURS

FITNESS LOG:

_____
_____
_____
_____

WATER TRACKER:

💧💧💧💧💧💧💧

FOOD LOG:

BREAKFAST:

LUNCH:

DINNER:

SNACKS:

DRINKS:

I AM GRATEFUL FOR:

_____
_____
_____
_____

AFFIRMATIONS:

_____
_____
_____
_____

THOUGHTS & REFLECTIONS:

_____
_____
_____
_____
_____
_____
_____
_____
_____
_____
_____
_____

DATE_____

TODAY I FEEL:

😖 🙁 😐 🙂 😊   _____
_____
_____

PREVIOUS NIGHT'S SLEEP QUALITY:

🙁 🙂 _____ HOURS

FITNESS LOG:
_____
_____
_____
_____
_____

WATER TRACKER:

💧💧💧💧💧💧💧

FOOD LOG:

BREAKFAST:
_____

LUNCH:
_____

DINNER:
_____

SNACKS:
_____

DRINKS:
_____

I AM GRATEFUL FOR:
___
___
___
___
___

AFFIRMATIONS:
___
___
___
___
___

THOUGHTS & REFLECTIONS:
___
___
___
___
___
___
___
___
___
___
___
___
___
___

DATE_____

TODAY I FEEL:

😣 🙁 😐 🙂 😊 _____
_____
_____

PREVIOUS NIGHT'S SLEEP QUALITY:

🙁 🙂 _____ HOURS

FITNESS LOG:
_____
_____
_____
_____
_____

WATER TRACKER:

💧💧💧💧💧💧💧

FOOD LOG:

BREAKFAST:
_____

LUNCH:
_____

DINNER:
_____

SNACKS:
_____

DRINKS:
_____

I AM GRATEFUL FOR:

_____
_____
_____
_____

AFFIRMATIONS:

_____
_____
_____
_____

THOUGHTS & REFLECTIONS:

_____
_____
_____
_____
_____
_____
_____
_____
_____
_____
_____
_____
_____

DATE_____

TODAY I FEEL:

😣 🙁 😐 🙂 😊 _____

PREVIOUS NIGHT'S SLEEP QUALITY:

🙁 🙂 _____ HOURS

FITNESS LOG:

_____
_____
_____
_____
_____

WATER TRACKER:

💧 💧 💧 💧 💧 💧 💧

FOOD LOG:

BREAKFAST:
_____

LUNCH:
_____

DINNER:
_____

SNACKS:
_____

DRINKS:
_____

I AM GRATEFUL FOR:

AFFIRMATIONS:

THOUGHTS & REFLECTIONS:

DATE _____

TODAY I FEEL:

😖 🙁 😐 🙂 😊 _____
_____
_____

PREVIOUS NIGHT'S SLEEP QUALITY:

🙁 🙂 _____ HOURS

FITNESS LOG:

_____
_____
_____
_____
_____

WATER TRACKER:

💧 💧 💧 💧 💧 💧 💧

FOOD LOG:

BREAKFAST: _____

LUNCH: _____

DINNER: _____

SNACKS: _____

DRINKS: _____

I AM GRATEFUL FOR:

AFFIRMATIONS:

THOUGHTS & REFLECTIONS:

DATE_____

TODAY I FEEL:

😫 ☹️ 😐 🙂 😊   _____
_____
_____
_____

PREVIOUS NIGHT'S SLEEP QUALITY:

☹️ 🙂 _____ HOURS

FITNESS LOG:
_____
_____
_____
_____
_____

WATER TRACKER:

💧💧💧💧💧💧💧

FOOD LOG:

BREAKFAST:
_____

LUNCH:
_____

DINNER:
_____

SNACKS:
_____

DRINKS:
_____

I AM GRATEFUL FOR:

_____
_____
_____
_____

AFFIRMATIONS:

_____
_____
_____
_____

THOUGHTS & REFLECTIONS:

_____
_____
_____
_____
_____
_____
_____
_____
_____
_____
_____
_____
_____

DATE_____

TODAY I FEEL:

😣 ☹️ 😐 🙂 😊 _____
_____
_____
_____

PREVIOUS NIGHT'S SLEEP QUALITY:

☹️ 🙂 _____ HOURS

FITNESS LOG:

_____
_____
_____
_____
_____

WATER TRACKER:

💧 💧 💧 💧 💧 💧 💧

FOOD LOG:

BREAKFAST: _____
_____

LUNCH: _____
_____

DINNER: _____
_____

SNACKS: _____
_____

DRINKS: _____
_____

I AM GRATEFUL FOR:

_____
_____
_____
_____

AFFIRMATIONS:

_____
_____
_____
_____
_____

THOUGHTS & REFLECTIONS:

_____
_____
_____
_____
_____
_____
_____
_____
_____
_____
_____
_____
_____
_____
_____

DATE_____

TODAY I FEEL:

😖 ☹️ 😐 🙂 😊 _____
_____
_____
_____

PREVIOUS NIGHT'S SLEEP QUALITY:

☹️ 🙂 _____ HOURS

FITNESS LOG:
_____
_____
_____
_____

WATER TRACKER:

💧💧💧💧💧💧💧

FOOD LOG:

BREAKFAST:
_____

LUNCH:
_____

DINNER:
_____

SNACKS:
_____

DRINKS:
_____

I AM GRATEFUL FOR:

AFFIRMATIONS:

THOUGHTS & REFLECTIONS:

DATE_____

TODAY I FEEL:

😣 ☹️ 😐 🙂 😊 _____
_____
_____
_____

PREVIOUS NIGHT'S SLEEP QUALITY:

☹️ 🙂 _____ HOURS

FITNESS LOG:
_____
_____
_____
_____
_____

WATER TRACKER:

◊ ◊ ◊ ◊ ◊ ◊ ◊

FOOD LOG:

BREAKFAST: _____

LUNCH: _____

DINNER: _____

SNACKS: _____

DRINKS: _____

I AM GRATEFUL FOR:

AFFIRMATIONS:

THOUGHTS & REFLECTIONS:

DATE_____

TODAY I FEEL:

😣 🙁 😐 🙂 😊   _____
                  _____
                  _____
                  _____

PREVIOUS NIGHT'S SLEEP QUALITY:

                🙁 🙂   _____ HOURS

FITNESS LOG:

_____
_____
_____
_____

WATER TRACKER:

💧 💧 💧 💧 💧 💧 💧

FOOD LOG:

BREAKFAST:
_____

LUNCH:
_____

DINNER:
_____

SNACKS:
_____

DRINKS:
_____

I AM GRATEFUL FOR:
___
___
___
___
___

AFFIRMATIONS:
___
___
___
___
___

THOUGHTS & REFLECTIONS:
___
___
___
___
___
___
___
___
___
___
___
___
___
___
___
___
___

DATE_____

TODAY I FEEL:

😫 🙁 😐 🙂 😊 _____

PREVIOUS NIGHT'S SLEEP QUALITY:

🙁 🙂 _____ HOURS

FITNESS LOG:

_____
_____
_____
_____
_____

WATER TRACKER:

💧 💧 💧 💧 💧 💧 💧

FOOD LOG:

BREAKFAST:

LUNCH:

DINNER:

SNACKS:

DRINKS:

I AM GRATEFUL FOR:

___

AFFIRMATIONS:

___

THOUGHTS & REFLECTIONS:

___

DATE _____

TODAY I FEEL:

😣 😕 😐 🙂 😊 _____

PREVIOUS NIGHT'S SLEEP QUALITY:

☹️ 🙂 _____ HOURS

FITNESS LOG:

_____
_____
_____
_____

WATER TRACKER:

💧💧💧💧💧💧💧

FOOD LOG:

BREAKFAST: _____

LUNCH: _____

DINNER: _____

SNACKS: _____

DRINKS: _____

I AM GRATEFUL FOR:

AFFIRMATIONS:

THOUGHTS & REFLECTIONS:

DATE_____

TODAY I FEEL:

😫 🙁 😐 🙂 😊 _____
_____
_____
_____

PREVIOUS NIGHT'S SLEEP QUALITY:

🙁 🙂 _____ HOURS

FITNESS LOG:

_____
_____
_____
_____
_____

WATER TRACKER:

💧💧💧💧💧💧💧

FOOD LOG:

BREAKFAST:
_____

LUNCH:
_____

DINNER:
_____

SNACKS:
_____

DRINKS:
_____

I AM GRATEFUL FOR:

AFFIRMATIONS:

THOUGHTS & REFLECTIONS:

DATE _____

TODAY I FEEL:

😣 ☹️ 😐 🙂 😊 _____
_____
_____

PREVIOUS NIGHT'S SLEEP QUALITY:

☹️ 🙂 _____ HOURS

FITNESS LOG:

_____
_____
_____
_____
_____

WATER TRACKER:

💧 💧 💧 💧 💧 💧 💧

FOOD LOG:

BREAKFAST:
_____

LUNCH:
_____

DINNER:
_____

SNACKS:
_____

DRINKS:
_____

I AM GRATEFUL FOR:

AFFIRMATIONS:

THOUGHTS & REFLECTIONS:

DATE_____

TODAY I FEEL:

😣 🙁 😐 🙂 😊 _____
_____
_____

PREVIOUS NIGHT'S SLEEP QUALITY:

🙁 🙂 _____ HOURS

FITNESS LOG:
_____
_____
_____
_____
_____

WATER TRACKER:

💧💧💧💧💧💧💧

FOOD LOG:

BREAKFAST: _____

LUNCH: _____

DINNER: _____

SNACKS: _____

DRINKS: _____

I AM GRATEFUL FOR:

AFFIRMATIONS:

THOUGHTS & REFLECTIONS:

DATE_____

TODAY I FEEL:

😫 🙁 😐 🙂 😊 _____
_____
_____
_____

PREVIOUS NIGHT'S SLEEP QUALITY:

🙁 🙂 _____ HOURS

FITNESS LOG:
_____
_____
_____
_____
_____

WATER TRACKER:

💧💧💧💧💧💧💧

FOOD LOG:

BREAKFAST:
_____

LUNCH:
_____

DINNER:
_____

SNACKS:
_____

DRINKS:
_____

I AM GRATEFUL FOR:

AFFIRMATIONS:

THOUGHTS & REFLECTIONS:

DATE_____

TODAY I FEEL:

😣 🙁 😐 🙂 😊   _____
_____
_____

PREVIOUS NIGHT'S SLEEP QUALITY:

🙁 🙂 _____ HOURS

FITNESS LOG:
_____
_____
_____
_____
_____

WATER TRACKER:

💧💧💧💧💧💧💧

FOOD LOG:

BREAKFAST: _____
_____

LUNCH: _____
_____

DINNER: _____
_____

SNACKS: _____
_____

DRINKS: _____
_____

I AM GRATEFUL FOR:

AFFIRMATIONS:

THOUGHTS & REFLECTIONS:

DATE_____

TODAY I FEEL:

😫 🙁 😐 🙂 😊 _____

PREVIOUS NIGHT'S SLEEP QUALITY:

🙁 🙂 _____ HOURS

FITNESS LOG:

_____
_____
_____
_____

WATER TRACKER:

💧💧💧💧💧💧💧

FOOD LOG:

BREAKFAST: _____

LUNCH: _____

DINNER: _____

SNACKS: _____

DRINKS: _____

I AM GRATEFUL FOR:

AFFIRMATIONS:

THOUGHTS & REFLECTIONS:

DATE_____

TODAY I FEEL:

😣 🙁 😐 🙂 😊 _____
_____
_____
_____

PREVIOUS NIGHT'S SLEEP QUALITY:

🙁 🙂 _____ HOURS

FITNESS LOG:

_____
_____
_____
_____
_____

WATER TRACKER:

💧 💧 💧 💧 💧 💧 💧

FOOD LOG:

BREAKFAST: _____

LUNCH: _____

DINNER: _____

SNACKS: _____

DRINKS: _____

I AM GRATEFUL FOR:

AFFIRMATIONS:

THOUGHTS & REFLECTIONS:

DATE _____

TODAY I FEEL:

😣 🙁 😐 🙂 😊   _____
_____
_____
_____

PREVIOUS NIGHT'S SLEEP QUALITY:

🙁 🙂   _____ HOURS

FITNESS LOG:

_____
_____
_____
_____
_____

WATER TRACKER:

◊ ◊ ◊ ◊ ◊ ◊ ◊

FOOD LOG:

BREAKFAST:
_____

LUNCH:
_____

DINNER:
_____

SNACKS:
_____

DRINKS:
_____

I AM GRATEFUL FOR:

AFFIRMATIONS:

THOUGHTS & REFLECTIONS:

DATE_____

TODAY I FEEL:

😣 🙁 😐 🙂 😊

PREVIOUS NIGHT'S SLEEP QUALITY:

🙁 🙂 _____ HOURS

FITNESS LOG:

WATER TRACKER:

💧💧💧💧💧💧💧

FOOD LOG:

BREAKFAST:

LUNCH:

DINNER:

SNACKS:

DRINKS:

I AM GRATEFUL FOR:

_____
_____
_____
_____

AFFIRMATIONS:

_____
_____
_____
_____

THOUGHTS & REFLECTIONS:

_____
_____
_____
_____
_____
_____
_____
_____
_____
_____
_____
_____
_____
_____

DATE_____

TODAY I FEEL:

😫 🙁 😐 🙂 😊 _____
_____
_____
_____

PREVIOUS NIGHT'S SLEEP QUALITY:

🙁 🙂 _____ HOURS

FITNESS LOG:
_____
_____
_____
_____
_____

WATER TRACKER:

💧💧💧💧💧💧💧

FOOD LOG:

BREAKFAST:
_____

LUNCH:
_____

DINNER:
_____

SNACKS:
_____

DRINKS:
_____

I AM GRATEFUL FOR:
_____
_____
_____
_____

AFFIRMATIONS:
_____
_____
_____
_____

THOUGHTS & REFLECTIONS:
_____
_____
_____
_____
_____
_____
_____
_____
_____
_____
_____
_____
_____

DATE_____

TODAY I FEEL:

😫 🙁 😐 🙂 😊

PREVIOUS NIGHT'S SLEEP QUALITY:

🙁 🙂 _____ HOURS

FITNESS LOG:

_____
_____
_____
_____
_____

WATER TRACKER:

💧 💧 💧 💧 💧 💧 💧

FOOD LOG:

BREAKFAST:
_____

LUNCH:
_____

DINNER:
_____

SNACKS:
_____

DRINKS:
_____

I AM GRATEFUL FOR:

AFFIRMATIONS:

THOUGHTS & REFLECTIONS:

DATE_____

TODAY I FEEL:

😖 🙁 😐 🙂 😊   _____
                 _____
                 _____
                 _____

PREVIOUS NIGHT'S SLEEP QUALITY:

🙁 🙂 _____ HOURS

FITNESS LOG:

_____
_____
_____
_____
_____

WATER TRACKER:

💧 💧 💧 💧 💧 💧 💧

FOOD LOG:

BREAKFAST:
_____

LUNCH:
_____

DINNER:
_____

SNACKS:
_____

DRINKS:
_____

I AM GRATEFUL FOR:

_____
_____
_____
_____

AFFIRMATIONS:

_____
_____
_____
_____

THOUGHTS & REFLECTIONS:

_____
_____
_____
_____
_____
_____
_____
_____
_____
_____
_____
_____
_____
_____

DATE _____

TODAY I FEEL:

😣 ☹ 😐 🙂 😊 _____
_____
_____
_____

PREVIOUS NIGHT'S SLEEP QUALITY:

☹ 🙂 _____ HOURS

FITNESS LOG:
_____
_____
_____
_____
_____

WATER TRACKER:

💧💧💧💧💧💧💧

FOOD LOG:

BREAKFAST: _____
_____

LUNCH: _____
_____

DINNER: _____
_____

SNACKS: _____
_____

DRINKS: _____
_____

I AM GRATEFUL FOR:

_____
_____
_____
_____
_____

AFFIRMATIONS:

_____
_____
_____
_____
_____

THOUGHTS & REFLECTIONS:

_____
_____
_____
_____
_____
_____
_____
_____
_____
_____
_____
_____
_____
_____
_____

DATE_____

TODAY I FEEL:

😖 🙁 😐 🙂 😊 _____

PREVIOUS NIGHT'S SLEEP QUALITY:

🙁 🙂 _____ HOURS

FITNESS LOG:

_____
_____
_____
_____
_____

WATER TRACKER:

💧 💧 💧 💧 💧 💧 💧

FOOD LOG:

BREAKFAST:
_____

LUNCH:
_____

DINNER:
_____

SNACKS:
_____

DRINKS:
_____

I AM GRATEFUL FOR:

_____
_____
_____
_____

AFFIRMATIONS:

_____
_____
_____
_____
_____

THOUGHTS & REFLECTIONS:

_____
_____
_____
_____
_____
_____
_____
_____
_____
_____
_____
_____
_____
_____

DATE_____

TODAY I FEEL:

😫 🙁 😐 🙂 😊

PREVIOUS NIGHT'S SLEEP QUALITY:

🙁 🙂 _____ HOURS

FITNESS LOG:

WATER TRACKER:

💧💧💧💧💧💧💧

FOOD LOG:

BREAKFAST:

LUNCH:

DINNER:

SNACKS:

DRINKS:

I AM GRATEFUL FOR:

AFFIRMATIONS:

THOUGHTS & REFLECTIONS:

DATE_____

TODAY I FEEL:

😣 🙁 😐 🙂 😊 _____

PREVIOUS NIGHT'S SLEEP QUALITY:

🙁 🙂 _____ HOURS

FITNESS LOG:

_____
_____
_____
_____
_____

WATER TRACKER:

💧💧💧💧💧💧💧

FOOD LOG:

BREAKFAST: _____

LUNCH: _____

DINNER: _____

SNACKS: _____

DRINKS: _____

I AM GRATEFUL FOR:

AFFIRMATIONS:

THOUGHTS & REFLECTIONS:

DATE _____

TODAY I FEEL:

😣 😟 😐 🙂 😊 _____
_____
_____
_____

PREVIOUS NIGHT'S SLEEP QUALITY:

😟 🙂 _____ HOURS

FITNESS LOG:
_____
_____
_____
_____
_____

WATER TRACKER:

◊ ◊ ◊ ◊ ◊ ◊ ◊

FOOD LOG:

BREAKFAST:
_____

LUNCH:
_____

DINNER:
_____

SNACKS:
_____

DRINKS:
_____

I AM GRATEFUL FOR:

_____
_____
_____
_____

AFFIRMATIONS:

_____
_____
_____
_____

THOUGHTS & REFLECTIONS:

_____
_____
_____
_____
_____
_____
_____
_____
_____
_____
_____
_____
_____

Made in the USA
Monee, IL
24 April 2025

c5f076e3-1c0a-4016-8320-a200579e2ba6R01